Turner Syndrome Diary

XOXOXOXO

XOXOXO   By: Amy

Tihlarik

Find Amy on Youtube ! Life of Amy Turner Syndrome

Amy has Patreon, You Now, Facebook, Twitter, and Instagram Also!!!!

Dedication: I dedicate this book to my mom and dad. The strength, love, kindness, compassion, and pure understanding of family really shows through in life. Especially when you are diagnosed with a condition not many people understand or care to understand for that matter. This goes out to them. Mom and dad, your love, honesty, and compassion does not and will not ever go unnoticed. Thanks for always being there for me, thanks for putting up with me, and thanks for giving me life. This ones for you. Xoxoxoxoxox

I love you as high as the sky, to the moon and back !!!! xoxoxoxoxoxoxoxo times infinity and beyond !!!!!! love, your "favorite kid"

Why am I writing this?????.....................

Sometimes in life you need to do something for you. Sometimes in life you need to do things that help you to fully understand why you are unlike other kids your age. Sometimes you need to try your hardest even on tough days, to put into perspective life. Even if your grammar and punctuation lack, even if you cannot find the right words to explain your feelings, even if you find yourself in a "dark place", why not continue to try till you "find the light". Keep trying till you find the inner happiness you have always been searching for. Keep trying till you find the inner happiness you DESERVE!!!.

For all the people still searching for their happiness, their place in the world, the understanding they so deeply are looking for, the understanding from others in a not understanding world. This diary is for you. Continue to be the superhero you are and always have been. Remember always, your worth it !!!!!!

Before we get started! On a Turner Syndrome Note!

Turner Syndrome always has been and will be super unique and complicated. To the world we are "NORMAL" to the world we are "like everyone else". But in all honesty, the depths of those statements hit us hard some days. The world is not all peaches and crème. The world is cruel, unfair, and sometimes just plain ridiculous. Having Turner Syndrome makes us superheroes, unique, strong, fabulous, and just plain AMAZING!!! Having Turner Syndrome and being able to sit and type this right now, makes me one of the 1% of people with Turner syndrome that survive till birth. Only 1%, yes not a typo, 1% of people with Turner Syndrome do NOT make it to birth. With that percentage and all that being said so far, I wrote this book. I wrote this book to look into my life, and my thoughts on having Turner Syndrome. I wrote this book to share the good and bad from the diagnosis through today as an adult. I wrote this in diary form, to share the ups and downs, the happy thoughts, the scared thoughts, the confusing thoughts, the "everything thoughts". As a diary, don't expect proper grammar,

punctuation, and that things will be 100% in "this makes sense form" this is the raw and real feelings that I went through. This diary is not my actual diary or my whole thoughts. This is a diary sharing the common thoughts in my head having Turner syndrome, but also, this is a diary from a Turner syndrome butterflies "common standpoint". I hope you enjoy my honesty. I hope you enjoy the general thoughts of having Turner Syndrome. I hope you enjoy the real powers and hope we all share having this unique diagnosis. I wrote this for the "happy butterflies", the "scared butterflies", the "hopeful butterflies", the "confused butterflies". I wrote this for you, enjoy! - Amy

XOXOXOXOXOXOXOXOXOXOXOXOXOXOXOXOXOXO XOXOXOXOX

XOXOXOXOXOXOXOXOXOXOXOXOXOXOXOXOXOXO XOXOXOXOX

XOXOXOXOXOXOXOXOXOXOXOXOXOXOXOXOXOXO XOXOXOXOX

ps! Remember the grammar, spelling, and punctuation is in the eyes of a child/teen, this does not in anyway dictate my abilities ⁇ hehe just so ya know! Wanted to make it the most relatable journey I could! xoxox lets begin the book.....................

November 1st, 1993

    Why am I here? My parents said it's because I don't grow at the rate other kids do. What's that even mean? I mean I am 9 years old, give me a break with the confusing talk lol jk hehe. Anyways, I just got this diary. I am gonna write in it cause I want to. Hehe

!!! because my parents think it will be a good idea. I don't agree. But, I will do it anyways. So, I sit here in this lobby trying to realize why being short is a crime. Why are my parents concerned about me being short? Why do I have to come to the docs anyways? Who knows I will wright again in a lil bit. Xoxoxo me!!!!

November 1st, 1993 still same day ugh what is life?

Omg what did I just go through? What just happened to me? this "dude" made my arm black and blue gee really !!!!!!! ugh I am not happy. He had to stick my arm 1,000,000 times and couldn't find the right spot to take my blood. Ugh ugh ugh !!!! I hate you hospital. I hate you blood sucking guy !!!!ok so apparently my parents say that now we wait for the results!!! The results?? What are we actually waiting for? No clue!!!! See ya soon !!!!!

November 10th, 1993

Why do I have to go back here !!!? I don't want to!!! You cant make me !!!! well......I guess you can make me !!!!...............................I am in this hospital waiting room yet again !!!! fuuuuuun !!!! NOT!!!!!! I guess I should be getting called back in soon ! talk to you when this silly business is over !!!!!!...........................continued !!!!! I got to watch Beauty And The Beast while this other person put some jelly stuff on my tummy. She said she was looking at my tummy and organs. Oh well I like this movie !!!!

November 10........Who care the date anymore !!!!!!!!

What is Turner Syndrome? Why did that doctor only talk to my parents? Why do I feel so confused like my life is weird or not even my own. Worst off, why did I have to sit in the waiting room again while the doctor only talked to my parents? That's rude, ...yip I said it, you doctor are the rudest person I have ever met. I had to have all the tests, not you !!!! why would you not tell me what's wrong with me? Y ai get it I am 9, but that doesn't mean you don't have to tell me what's wrong with me. Once I got to go back in they talked to me like I knew all the big words the doctor was talking about. uhhhhhh no, I don't get it doc nice try. Oh well, I will ask my parents later I guess !!!!!!! c-ya soon diary -me

November 9th, 1993 later that day at the house!!!!

I guess Turner syndrome is when you need shots to help you grow taller like your friends. I don't care, I have always been short. Whats the difference if I am short forever???? I see no difference. But mom and pop tell me I need them and that's that !!!! I hate shots, I hate that doctor, I hate this Turner Syndrome, whatever Turner

Syndrome is !!!! the doctor was just talking about X this and X that !!! really doctor, I don't understand this X talk. Oh well, I hate X's and I hate Shots.....I Hate you Turner Syndrome !!!......Whatever you are. But I guess, if mom and dad say it's a good thing I believe them. When do the needles start ? !!!! ahhhhhhhhhhh SEND HELP SOS !!!!!!!! #notgoingto likethis #saveme #goawayturnersyndrome

November 20th, 1993

Are you kidding me? My MOTHER gives me the shots!!!! Are you insain doctor? Have you lost the last of your marbles? I don't need answer this hurts. My mom is more scared of giving me the shots than I am of taking them. Ugh, how long does this go on for? Nobody ever told me how long this has to go on for. This is torture! I don't want shots anymore !!! I wanna be a normal kid !!!! Im done writing today .... Peace out !!

November 22nd, 1993

Bruises, I hate bruises. These Shots give me Bruises ! I want the pain to go away.... I want the bruises to go away. Someone make me normal so the bruises from the needles and shots can go away.!!!!! No takers ? L(kk.............I was told by mom and dad the shots will help me grow and I will finally be the same height as others, I will finally be normal !!!! hmmmmm !! why do I have a feeling somebodies lying to me

?.......we will see!!! #shotssuck
inpainandnothappy-me

NO DATE FOR YOU DIARY !!! (mad
at you diary) 1993 still

   I have to go have checkups every 3-
4 months at this place for .....whats the
word endocrinology. I have to see the
doctor for that, mom calls him an
endocrinologist or whatever. HE I guess
is the one checking up on me and my
Turner Syndrome now. He is nice
enough and he doesn't make me take
9,000,000 things of blood each time I
go. He only takes like 2-3 things of
blood each time I go. I guess that's not
too bad I suppose. These checkups get
easier and easier. I wont write every
checkup cause why?....they do the same

thing each time. Height, weight, a normal checkup. That's boring, that's all they do each time haha ....Wonder when I don't have to go to that place at all lol ....see ya later !!!!

-Still 1993

    I wanna talk school for a bit. Why, because school is so hard for me. I mean, I can read from a young age, I can write, but math is so hard for me, I don't understand why it has to be soooooo hard, I don't know what I did to deserve this treatment by my teacher. She is mad at me. I write this today of all days because she got mad at me. She told me she knew I understood the math problems, and I wasn't allowed to go to recess if I didn't finish the problems. She claimed, "I know you can do it", "I know you know this stuff". To be honest diary, I really didn't understand. I don't get why she doesn't understand that I don't understand. This stuff is hard for me. My mom says it's a TS thing. I don't know if it is. Honestly diary, when it comes to math, it's like .... someone can show me and explain to me lots of different times how to do a problem. The problem is, the more ways I am shown, the more times and I explained a problem, my brain says nope nope nope !! it's not gonna happen. My brain just freezes, I just do not get it. Math is sooo hard for me diary and I just needed to vent. I hope one day a teacher can help me to the point that I ACTUALLY get it and understand. Who knows! – just me venting! -talk soon, -me

1994 !!@!! On a Monday Yahoo !!!

I only had to see the specialist for about a year !!!! yahoo I am so excited !!!!!!! now I don't have to go every 3-4 months I cannot believe it!!!! The doctor said I am doing good, every check up is good, and ya I am feeling more and more like a normal person now no more shots either I took them a year and nooooooooo more I don't care if I am tall!!! I don't care if I am tall!!! I don't care if I am tall !!! that's my new mantra by the time I am the same height as everyone else I won't care what people say about me nope I won't moms on bored me stopping them too yahoooo!!!!!! He (the doc) said I will just need to go back when I am older for some hormone stuff !!! don't know what that is totally but I don't care !!!!! I am FREEEEEEEE!!! I am a normal kid now !!!!! yahooooooooooooooooo! Love you diary ! xoxoxo -me

July 1st, 1995

    Hi again, a few years have went by because I had nothing to say. To be honest diary, I was mad at you. I am not mad at you anymore, buttttt

!!!!.....I am 11 now. I was mad at you because you didn't help me when I needed answers to my questions about this Turner Syndrome stuff. Its okay now, I better get it and I wont be mad at you anymore. I realize Turner Syndrome doesn't go away. But you wanna know one cool thing about it? Even though it wont go away, I still feel like a normal kid so that's good. I still don't have a lot of friends, and a few kids pick on me still and call me short and other short names but its ok, I don't like mean people anyways. Don't worry diary I I will ignore it.....well, I will try to ignore it lol............love you diary !! xoxoxo -me see ya soon xooxoxo -memememe

I am 14 still soooooo........ ! and I am infertile !!!! No date for you ! we need to focus on the more important issues at hand diary than the date and year it is ....

   While I was thinking I new everything there was to know about Turner Syndrome, I was left out of a few key elements in my life !!! like the fact that people with Turner Syndrome cannot have kids of their own! What!!! !@!$%^ how and why did this happen? Now what am I going to do? what am I going to tell people? What am I going to tell my boyfriends of the future? Is this something you even tell people? How do I know? All I know is I am heartbroken, scared, sad, crushed, defeated, and ya.....being a teenager sucks !!!! I suppose one positive about it all is I am still young enough to have a lot of time to think about all of this and what I want to be when I grow up. I would like to know now at the age of 14, however I don't think I am in the right age bracket still to think about the future in this magnitude. So, I am leaving this as a " cliffhanger" of my life. What will be will be. God grant me the serenity......to accept the things I cannot change ~!!!,...I guess. Xoxoxo - me

Sometime in March, 2000

You lied Diary, You are a liar so I threw you under the bed!!!! I wanted to pull you back out just to yell at you !!!! You were supposed to help me understand. You were supposed to help me and tell me what to do to get friends, you were supposed to help me make the bullies go away but you didn't !!!!! how dare you !!!! anyways I figured it out on my own no thanks to you !!!!! I pulled you out just to yell and ya YELL !!! I wanna yell loud and clear because you never helped me back then !!! I had no friends and a lot of bullies!!!!! Yup they called me names, put their arms on me and said I was an "arm rest" etc....yadda yadda yadda.......so guess what? I pulled you back out to tell you my life is good now!!!! NO THANKS TO YOU DIARY

!!!! five years later I had to figure out all the confusion on my own !!!! all this mess alone !!!! so ya

....
.................i'm not mad anymore but yes, My best friend is HOLLY she's the best. We hang out all the time and I love her xoxoxo we hang out everyday and life is good FINALLY !!!! I finally at the age of 16 feel like I belong. I finally feel like life is picking up for me !!!!!!!! I finally am happy.

March 15th, 2000

　　What changed in my life you may ask? Well I decided ON MY OWN ! I wasn't going to allow people to pick on me, be mean to me, let people treat me bad !!! I decided on my own I was not going to allow people to make me shy and not put myself out their in my now high school years !!!! no way no way. I was not going to be the shy and Quiet person I had always been. I was not going to allow people to dictate the person I need to be or should be. I want friends dangit haha. I also want a boyfriend too one day.....one day lol........I can wait longer on that last one I think though hehe......I have another Turner Syndrome appointment next week or something. I will keep you updated ok....Something about estrogen and getting boobs haha, my moms words not mine lol.............see ya soon. !!!!!

March, 2002

I am 18 now yahoo !!!!!!!!!! my the time goes so fast I cannot even believe it !!!! I am loving my life and everyone in it. I have a boyfriend now and I finally feel like a normal person !!!!!! I can't explain to you how good it feels to have life be exactly where it is supposed to be. The estrogen I was on for a small amount of time I felt like it wasn't working. I dunno if that's how it should feel or not. Buuuuuut, I don't care. My boyfriends name is Bruce. He treats me like I'm a normal human, I love it and I love him. He brought up marriage already!!! Are you kidding me, nooooooooooo!!! Why would I do that when life for me is just beginning. I don't think so hunny! Hehe. It is however super duper to have a boyfriend for the first time in my whole life. I hope I can keep him around for a bit lol. I have so many feelings inside, and diary let me tell ya they are the good feelings. The feelings of belonging, acceptance, having my own group, all of it, it rocks!. Honestly diary, I think this is going to be one of my last entries for a while. I don't want you to feel bad, I just want You to know that I am a young adult now. I have many other things I need to focus on, and ya, none of my other friends have diaries still. I never told anyone I have you still, because that's weird. I am sorry diary I love you. I will try to write again soon! Xoxoxox – me

The year 2003-

What !!! another two years has gone by diary. I am sorry I haven't written in years. I have let my adult life consume me in all the best and worst ways possible. I hope you understand. I get that journaling is very therapeutic, yes, I said journaling not writing in a diary. I apologize anyways. I worked at Toys R us for a bit. I loved it. Me and the original boyfriend broke up, irreconcilable differences, and I now must move yet again. I am heartbroken and sad to leave the life I now have made for myself. Why oh why? I don't know how this will be. I do not even want to imagine the thought of leaving once again to a new place and starting over again. I shall see what happens now. I will talk again soon after this move and all the feelings, I am feeling is over. Ps, Sorry I haven't been writing the exact dates just the years, I think it more important to have and add years than the actual dates haha !! ok by diary.....

-me.....

-Still 2003

I have now graduated from high school. Yes, a few weeks after the graduation is when I found out we were moving yet again. I am moving in with my sister because ......I want to !!! I don't want to start over !!! oh well, I am an adult now and these are adult things. Get over it, get over yourself, deal with it, adult. These are my mantras as of recently. -me

-The year is 2005

WOW! I like it here. I have a good job, a very good friend that I adore and WILL be my very best friend forever I can feel it !!!! and life is "boring". I have now an adult life, with adult responsibilities, and I have a new boyfriend. He is a gem. We will see how long this lasts, but YOLO (you only live once). Work consumes a lot of my life, but I am happy to be a productive member of society!!! #ADULTING -me

-The year is 2009

Finally, college bound !!! oh my!! I am a nontraditional student by all rights, but I don't care. I finally want to make something more of my life. I finally want to do something that makes me very proud. I can and WILL succeed !!! wish me luck!!

-Still 2009

College math is so tough. I am bound and determined to do it. I just really wish I could explain to math teacher to make him understand my past. I want him to know my track record with math issues. I just want one teacher to understand and help me through math once and for all. Am I gonna do it?......I hope so!!!

CONTINUED...........I failed math class once ugh !!! but I am happy to announce, I passed it the second time. I was so very upset diary; I mean sad. I just had to tell myself stop it !!!! just do it again, you know the stuff now, one more try. OMG! One more try worked. I cannot believe diary that I didn't give up !!!! I have never been so proud of myself !!! I am the happiest I have ever been! if I can tackle a lifelong struggle like math, I can tackle anything!!!! #bringitonmath #iwinmath xoxoxox - me

- Year 2011

I am 27 now !!! and today I graduated college!!! Of all the things I am proud of in my life, this tops the list. I have never been so happy in my life. I am the type of happy today at the age of 27, that a little kid getting their training wheels off and taking their first spin of real freedom is !! that mind blowing happy, that a tornado can swoop through and I'm still gonna be smiling happy, the nothing can break my stride happy !!! I am the cant put into words ever type of happy. I am eternally proud of myself!!! I DID IT !! I MADE IT!!!! LIFE IS GOOD !! #collegewarrior

-Year 2013

I am 29 now !!! I need a family of my own. I need the missing pieces. I told myself I was happy being alone. I told my self my whole life to be happy with what god gave me. I told myself to get a job using my college degrees, get a dog, and be happy. I never was a good listener haha. Today I started the process to do foster care. I have never been more scared or terrifies in my whole life. I have never had so many questions, thoughts, and emotions in my body ever!!!! I hope this process really completes my life, completes my happiness, and makes all the trials and tribulations of life worth it. I am going to do it, I am going to do it, I am going to make it. I deserve this!!!!! I love you diary, thanks for always being my listening ear. I hope one day I can look back at all these things I have went through and know it was all for a purpose. Xooxoxoxox I love you -me

-Year 2014

I did it!!!! OMG diary I did it !!!! I just got licensed to be a foster parent!!!! I am crying hysterically writing this because I have never been so alive. I never knew what this could feel like. Its like 1,000 weights have been on my back this whole time and now it feels right. Life feels right, everything is right!!!!.... I have no words....i have no words, i.....OMG...!!! I am goanna be a mom!!!! Diary, ... I AM GOING TO BE A MOM!

-Year 2014 Still

I got the call today, the call I have waited my whole life for. Dreams do come true. I am getting placed with a foster child. I cannot tell you how deep those words mean to my heart. I must prepare; I have to finish up my last-minute stuff. .....I am a mom !!!!! omg !!!! MOM...I will never get sick of hearing that word!

xoxoxoxoxox -me

the year still 2014-

Today I made my foster kid a diary of the process of foster care, me waiting for him, my journey, my life, my story. I put it in the pages of the Dr. Seuss book "oh The Places You'll Go". I hope he will find comfort reading the entries when he is older. Thank you so much for listening diary. I am thankful you gave me all these years of a listening ear !! I hope you know how much I needed this diary at many points of good and bad in my life. I will forever be grateful to you !!!! thanks for believing in me when I didn't believe in myself !!!! xoxox on to our next adventures of life...... until we talk again diary

.... Love,

- me xoxoxox

- THE END.......OOPS, I MEANT
....TO BE CONTINUED
....

<u>Conclusion from the Author Amy Tihlarik !</u>

As this diary comes to an end, I want to say thank you to so many people in my "real life" that deserve so much gratitude for helping me find myself when I was lost throughout the years!!! Thank you all for believing in me when I honestly didn't believe in myself. And thank you for continuing to be there for me and my sons today! xoxoxox you know who you are!!!

xoxo love, Amy